THE ESSENTIAL AIR FRYER COOKBOOK FOR BEGINNERS

From Simple Breakfast to Lunch and Dinner Meals

Hollie McCarthy RDN

INTRODUCTION

Welcome to the air fryer guide!

The air fryer is one of the most impressive and useful inventions of the decade. With this machine, you can reduce the amount of grease you consume from traditional dishes and snacks such as chicken nuggets and French fries. Goes without saying that cooking time is considerably reduced!

It is a multi-cooker that performs more than functions. The air fryer enables you to cook a wide variety of dishes including meat, fish, eggs, grain, poultry, beans, cakes, yogurt and vegetables etc. What Serves: it exceptional is because you can use different cooking programs such as a steamer, rice cooker, sauté pan, and even a warming pot, thus saving more time, money, and space than buying any other kitchen appliances.

The Air fryer Serves: as a multi-use programmable appliance can help create easy, fast and flavorful recipes with the ability to apply different cooking settings all in one pot. It was developed by Canadian technology experts seeking to be the ultimate kitchen mate, from stir-frying, pressure cooking, slow cooking and yogurt and cake making. It was created to serve as a one-stop shop to allow home cooks prepare a tasty meal with the press of a button. You can cook almost everything in this fryer.

The air fryer uses an ingenious combination of both Directions, differing from the convection oven because heat circulates everywhere (vice rising to the top) through the fan, and not through the turbo because there is typically no heating element in the top of a fryer from where the heat comes out. They use electrical energy to create their heat; a lot of power!

Many people still have their doubts regarding the importance of this machine, and what a healthy alternative it can be. Despite its popularity, in some regions it has not yet reached the peak of its use. It is very likely that in a short time new brands will emerge in other regions and the air fryer will grow in popularity across the nation.

The use of this tool consists of cooking something without boiling the product in oil or fat. At most, the maximum oil needed by the air fryer is a tablespoon, which is used to prevent the food from sticking and forming an overdone crust.

What is an air fryer?

An air fryer works with "fast air technology." This means that there is a highspeed circulation of hot air that cocoons the food you cook.

During this process, the air fryer prepares the food evenly, all the while giving it a "fried" taste and texture without ever actually having to fry anything in grease.

While many people and regions near and far are familiar with this tool, the electric fryer is even crossing the waters. They are even found commonly in Europe and Australia!

The air fryer is similar in concept to a convection oven or a turbo grill, although the fryer still differs slightly from both appliances. Convection ovens and turbo broilers depend on different heating Directions and are often larger and bulkier appliances to use when cooking your food.

In this book, we will explore the variety of easy delicious dishes you can cook with your air fryer. We will explore a wide variety of dishes, from breakfast to dinner, soups to stews, desserts to appetizers, meat to beef, side dishes to vegetables and use a healthy ingredient in the process. The vast majority of the recipes can be prepared and served in less than 45 minutes. Each recipe is written with the exact cooking Directions and ingredients required to prepare dishes that will satisfy and nourish you. Once you try the delish dishes in this cookbook, you and your air fryer are sure to become inseparable too.

It's important to think outside the box when it comes to trying out recipes in your air fryer. From roasted vegetables to empanadas, to baked eggs and vegan brownies, there's an option for everyone when you use your air fryer.

This cookbook is for people who want to create tasty dishes without spending all day in the kitchen. Most of the recipes can be prepared in 15 minutes or less. And most of them can be on the table in under an hour. With today's busy lifestyles, I know this is important to most of you.

In keeping with the latest health trends and diets, the recipes also include complete nutrition information. As a plus, there are recipes for those on a Vegan Diet as well as Mediterranean diet.

Let's delve in!

Bacon and Eggs for Breakfast

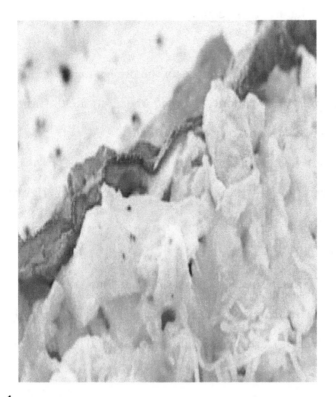

Serves: 1

Ingredients

- 4 strips of thick-sliced bacon
- 2 small eggs
- Salt and black pepper, to taste
- Oil spray for greasing ramekins

Directions

1. Take 2 ramekins and grease them with oil spray.

2. Crack eggs in a bowl and season it salt and black pepper.

3. Divide the egg mixture between two ramekins.

4. Preheat the unit by selecting AIR FRY mode for 3 minutes at 325 degrees F.

5. Select START/PAUSE to begin the preheating process.

6. Once preheating is done, put the ramekin inside the bottom of the air fryer basket, and bacon on the side.

7. Put the basket inside the unit.

8. Now set it to AIR FRY mode at 400 degrees F, for 12 minutes.

9. Press start to begin the cooking.

10. Once done, serve and enjoy.

Variation Tip: Use butter for greasing ramekins

Nutritional Information Per Serving: Calories131 | Fat 10g| Sodium 187mg | Carbs0.6 g | Fiber 0g | Sugar 0.6g | Protein 10.7

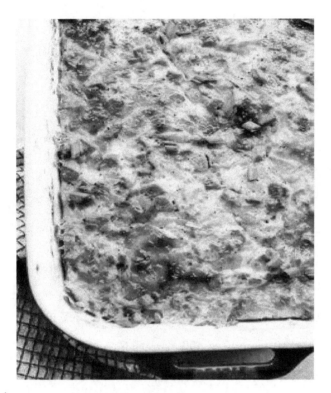

Serves: 4

Ingredients

- 1 pound of beef sausage, grounded

- 1/4 cup diced white onion

- 1 diced green bell pepper

- 8 whole eggs, beaten

- ½ cup Colby jack cheese, shredded

- ¼ teaspoon of garlic salt

- Oil spray, for greasing

Directions

1. Take a bowl and add ground sausage to it.

2. Add in the diced onions, bell peppers, eggs and whisk it well.

3. Then season it with garlic salt.

4. Spray the basket of the air fryer with oil spray.

5. Preheat the unit by selecting AIR FRY mode for 5 minutes at 325 degrees F.

6. Select START/PAUSE to begin the preheating process.

7. Once preheating is done, place the mixture inside the basket; remember to remove the crisper plate.

8. Top the mixture with cheese.

9. Now, turn ON the Air Fryer and select AIR FRY mode, and set the time to 10 minutes at 390 degrees F.

10. Once the cooking cycle completes, take out, and serve.

11. Serve and enjoy.

Serving Suggestion: Serve it with sour cream

Variation Tip: Use turkey sausages instead of beef sausages.

Nutritional Information Per Serving: Calories 699| Fat 59.1g | Sodium 1217 mg | Carbs 6.8g | Fiber 0.6g| Sugar 2.5g | Protein33.1g

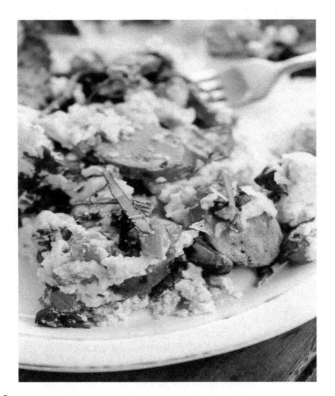

Serves: 2

Ingredients

- 4 sausage links, raw and uncooked

- 4 eggs, uncooked

- 1 tablespoon of green onion

- 1 tablespoon of chopped tomatoes

- Salt and black pepper, to taste

- 2 tablespoons of milk

- Oil spray, for greasing

Directions

1.   Take a bowl and whisk eggs in it.

2.   Then pour milk, and add onions and tomatoes.

3.   Whisk it all well.

4.   Now season it with salt and black pepper.

5.   Take one cake pan, that fits inside the air fryer and grease it with oil spray.

6.   Pour the omelet into the greased cake pans.

7.   Slice the sausages in round shapes and top them on eggs.

8.   Preheat the unit by selecting AIR FRY mode for 3 minutes at 325 degrees F.

9.   Select START/PAUSE to begin the preheating process.

10.   Once preheating is done, put the cake pan inside the unit.

11.   Select bake function of air fryer, and set the timer to 12 minutes at 310 degrees F.

12.   Once the cooking cycle completes, serve by transferring it to plates.

13.   Enjoy hot as a delicious breakfast.

Serving Suggestion: Serve it with toasted bread slices

Variation Tip: Use almond milk if like non-dairy milk

Nutritional Information Per Serving: Calories 240 | Fat 18.4g| Sodium 396mg | Carbs 2.8g | Fiber0.2g | Sugar 2g | Protein 15.6g

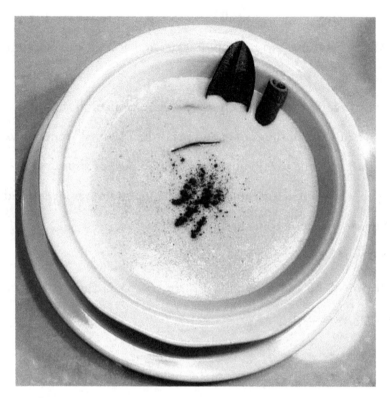

Serves: 6

Ingredients

- 6 cups water

- 1 ¼ cups coconut milk

- 1 ¼ cups yellow cornmeal, fine

- 2 ½ sticks cinnamon

- 1 ¼ teaspoons vanilla extract

- ¾ teaspoon coconut flakes

- ¾ cup sweetened condensed milk

Directions

1. Add 5 cups of water and all the coconut milk to the Air Fryer.
2. Mix the cornmeal with 1 cup of water and add the mixture to the pot.
3. Stir in vanilla extract, coconut flakes, and cinnamon sticks.
4. Secure the lid of the cooker and press the "Manual" function key.
5. Adjust the time to 6 minutes and cook at high pressure.
6. After the beep, release the pressure naturally and remove the lid.
7. Stir in sweetened condensed milk.
8. Serve and enjoy.

Nutrition Values (Per Serving): Calories: 253, Carbohydrate: 46.2g, Protein: 6.9g, Fat: 3.1g

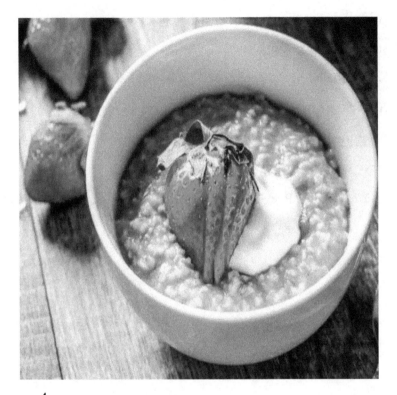

Serves: 4

Ingredients

- 2 cups old-fashioned oats

- 2 ¼ cups water

- 2 ¼ cups milk

- ½ teaspoon salt

- ½ teaspoon ground cinnamon

- ¼ cup sugar

- 8 strawberries, chopped

Directions

1. Add all the listed ingredients to the Air Fryer. Save a few strawberry slices for garnishing.

2. Secure the lid of the cooker and press the "Multigrain option."

3. Adjust the time to 6 minutes and let it cook.

4. After the beep, release the pressure naturally and remove the lid.

5. Serve with the chopped strawberries on top.

Nutrition Values (Per Serving): Calories: 436| Carbohydrate: 75g| Protein: 14.7g| Fat: 8g

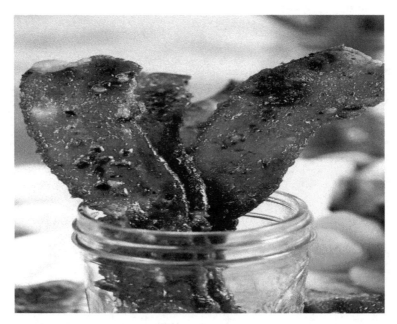

Serves: 4

Ingredients:

- 1 pound bacon, sliced

- 1/2 tsp ground paprika

- 1/2 tsp chili pepper

- Salt and pepper to taste

Directions:

1. Preheat your cooking machine to 145 degrees F.

2. Mix the ingredients thoroughly but carefully, making sure the bacon slices are evenly covered with spices.

3. Place the ingredients in the vacuum bag.

4. Seal it, set the timer for 9 hours.

5. Preheat the skillet and roast each slice on both sides for 10-15 seconds.

6. Serve hot.

Nutrition per serving: Calories: 360| Protein: 12 g| Fats: 35 g| Carbs: 9 g

Broccoli in Oyster Sauce

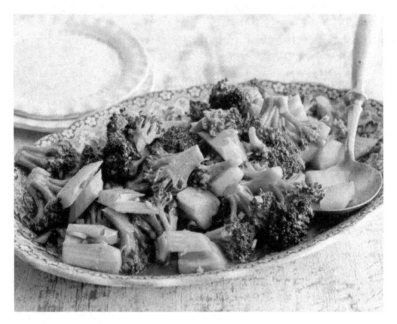

Serves: 4

Ingredients:

- 2 cups broccoli florets

- 1 tbsp oyster sauce

- 2 tbsp olive oil

- Salt and pepper to taste

- 1 garlic clove, minced

Directions:

1. Preheat your cooking machine to 183 degrees F.

2. Mix the ingredients and place them in the vacuum bag.

3. Seal the bag and put it in the water bath, setting the timer for 35 minutes.

4. Carefully mix with the minced garlic clove before serving.

Nutrition per serving: Calories: 160| Protein: 3 g| Fats: 14 g| Carbs: 9 g

Button Mushrooms & Parmesan

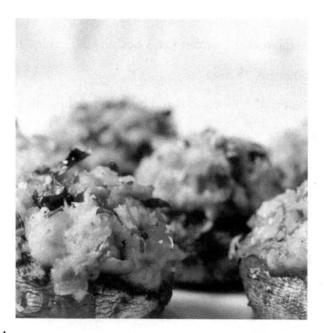

Serves: 4

Ingredients:

- 1 pound button mushrooms, coarsely chopped

- 4 tbsp olive oil

- 1 garlic clove, minced

- 1 cup Parmesan cheese, shredded

- 1/4 cup dry white wine

- 2 tbsp black truffle oil

- Salt and pepper to taste

Directions:

1. Set your cooking device to 180 degrees F.

2. Mix the mushrooms with olive oil, sprinkle with salt and pepper and place them in the vacuum bag. Seal the bag removing the air.

3. Set the timer for 35 minutes.

4. Heat a skillet, add the cooked and drained mushrooms and pour over the white wine.

5. Simmer until the liquid evaporates.

6. Serve sprinkled with the truffle oil and topped with grated Parmesan cheese.

Nutrition per serving:: Calories: 280| Protein: 10 g| Fats: 25 g| Carbs: 7 g

Brussel Sprouts Teriyaki

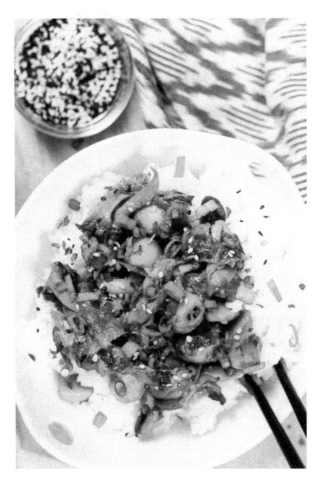

Serves: 4

Ingredients:

- pound Brussel sprouts
- tbsp Teriyaki sauce
- 2 tbsp olive oil
- Salt and pepper to taste

- 1 garlic clove, minced

Directions:

1. Set your cooking device to 183 degrees F.
2. In a salad bowl, mix the ingredients and place them in the vacuum bag. Seal the bag removing the air.
3. Put the bag into the water bath and set the cooking time for 35 minutes.
4. Carefully mix the sprouts with the minced garlic clove before serving.

Nutrition per serving: Calories: 159 | Protein: 3 g | Fats: 13 g | Carbs: 8 g

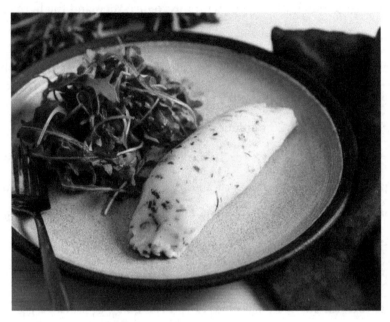

Serves: 2

Ingredients:

- 3 eggs
- 1 tbsp melted butter
- 1/2 tbsp tarragon, minced
- 1/2 tbsp rosemary, minced
- 1 tbsp plain yogurt
- Salt and pepper to taste
- 1 tbsp parsley, finely chopped (for serving)
- 1 tbsp grated Parmesan (for serving)

Directions:

1. Preheat your cooking machine to 165 degrees F.

2. In a large bowl, whisk eggs with the yogurt, then add the herbs and mix again.

3. Pour the ingredients into the vacuum bag, seal it, and put it in the water bath.

4. Set the timer for 20 minutes.

5. After cooking the eggs for 10 minutes, carefully remove them and press them into the shape of an omelet. Cook for 10 more minutes.

6. Remove the omelet from the bag, wait till it cools down, chop into the portions and serve as a starter garnished with the chopped parsley and grated Parmesan.

Nutrition per serving: Calories: 140| Protein: 15 g| Fats: 12 g| Carbs: 1.7 g

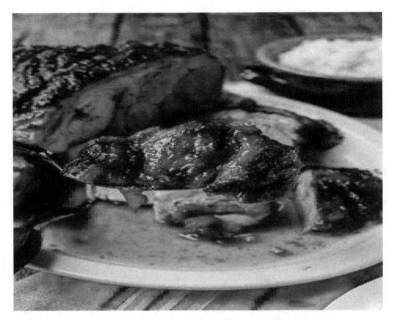

Serves: 2

Sauce Ingredients

- 4 tablespoons of soy sauce

- ¼ cup red wine

- 2 tablespoons of oyster sauce

- ¼ tablespoons of hoisin sauce

- ¼ cup honey

- ¼ cup brown sugar

- Pinch of salt

- Pinch of black pepper

- 1 teaspoon of ginger garlic, paste

- 1 teaspoon of five-spice powder

Other Ingredients

- 1.5 pounds of pork shoulder, sliced

Directions

1. Take a bowl and mix all the ingredients listed under sauce ingredients.

2. Transfer half of it to a saucepan and let it cook for 10 minutes.

3. Set it aside.

4. Let the pork marinate in the remaining sauce for 2 hours.

5. Afterward, put the pork slices in the basket and set it to AIRFRY mode 450 degrees for 25 minutes.

6. Make sure the internal temperature is above 160 degrees F once cooked.

7. If not add a few more minutes to the overall cooking time.

8. Once done, take it out and baste it with prepared sauce.

9. Serve and Enjoy.

Nutritional Information Per Serving: Calories 1239| Fat 73 g| Sodium 2185 mg | Carbs 57.3 g | Fiber 0.4g| Sugar53.7 g | Protein 81.5 g

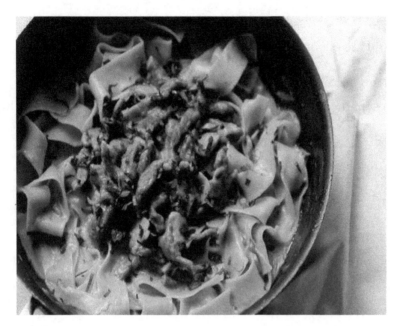

Serves: 6

Ingredients

- 1½ lbs beef stew meat

- 1½ tablespoons olive oil

- 1½ tablespoons garlic

- ¾ cup diced onions

- 1½ teaspoons salt

- 2 cups mushroom, chopped

- 1 cup water

- 1½ teaspoons black pepper

- ¾ cup sour cream

Directions

1. Select the 'sauté' function on the Air Fryer.

2. Add the oil, onions, and garlic. Cook for 3 minutes.

3. Add the remaining ingredients, except the sour cream.

4. Secure the lid and set the cooker on 'manual' for 20 minutes at high pressure.

5. After the beep, 'natural release' the steam and remove the lid after20 minutes.

6. Stir in the sour cream and serve.

Nutrition Values (Per Serving): Calories: 317| Carbohydrate: 4.4g| Protein: 36.4g| Fat: 16.6g

Eastern Lamb Stew

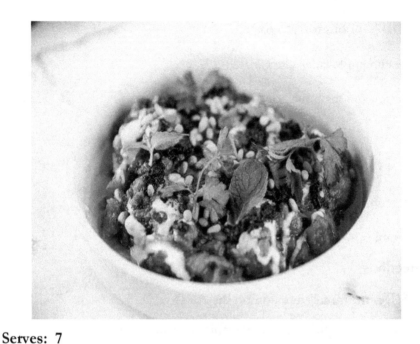

Serves: 7

Ingredients

- 4 tablespoons olive oil

- 1 (½ -1¾) lb lamb stew meat

- 2 onions, diced

- 8 garlic cloves, chopped

- 2 teaspoons salt and pepper

- 2 teaspoons cumin

- 2 teaspoons coriander

- 2 teaspoons turmeric,

- 2 teaspoons cinnamon

- 1 teaspoon chili flakes

- 4 tablespoons tomato paste

- ½ cup apple cider vinegar

- 4 tablespoons honey or brown sugar

- 2½ cups chicken broth

- 2 (15 oz.) cans chickpeas, rinsed and drained

- ½ cup raisins, chopped

- 2 tablespoons fresh cilantro to garnish, chopped

Directions

1. Select the 'sauté' function on the Air Fryer.

2. Add the oil, garlic, and all the spices. Sauté for 4 minutes.

3. Stir in all the remaining ingredients and secure the lid.

4. Switch the cooker to the 'meat stew' mode for 1 hour 15 minutes.

5. After the beep, 'natural release' the steam and remove the lid.

6. Stir the stew and serve with fresh cilantro on top.

Nutrition Values (Per Serving): Calories: 1010| Carbohydrate: 87.2g| Protein: 65.4g| Fat: 44.2g

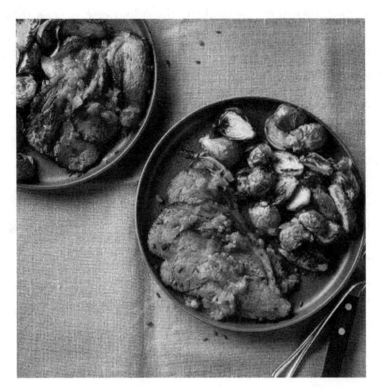

Serves: 8

Ingredients

- 6 lbs beef top sirloin steak

- 4 teaspoons garlic powder

- 8 cloves garlic, minced

- 1 cup butter

- Salt and pepper to taste

Directions

1. Select the 'sauté' function on the Air Fryer.

2. Add the butter to the pot and add the sirloin steaks. Cook for 5 minutes. Let the meat brown on each side.

3. Stir in all the remaining ingredients and secure the lid.

4. Switch the cooker to the 'meat stew' mode and cook for 30 minutes.

5. After the beep, 'natural release' the steam and remove the lid.

6. Serve hot.

Nutrition Values (Per Serving): Calories: 865 | Carbohydrate: 2g | Protein: 103.9g | Fat: 44.3g

Lamb Meat Balls

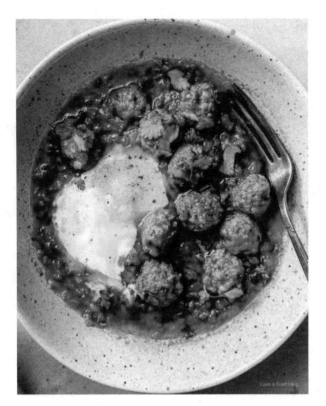

Serves: 3

Ingredients

- ¾ lbs ground lamb meat

- Salt and freshly ground black pepper, to taste

- 2 small tomatoes, chopped roughly

- ½ small yellow onion, chopped roughly

- ½ cup sugar-free tomato sauce

- ¼ teaspoon red pepper flakes, crushed

- 2 garlic cloves, peeled

- 5 mini bell peppers, seeded and halved

- ½ tablespoon olive oil

- 1 teaspoon adobo seasoning*

Directions

1. In a bowl, combine the lamb meat with the adobo seasoning*.

2. Prepare small meatballs out of this mixture.

3. Set the cooker to the 'sauté' mode and add the oil to it.

4. Add the meatballs to the hot oil and cook until they turn golden brown.

5. Transfer the meatballs to a separate bowl.

6. Add all the remaining ingredients to the pot and secure the lid.

7. Switch the cooker to the 'meat stew' mode and cook for 35 minutes.

8. After the beep, 'natural release the steam and remove the lid.

9. Use an immersion blender to blend the vegetable mix.

10. Stir in the meatballs, garnish with herbs, and serve hot.

Nutrition Values (Per Serving): Calories: 445| Carbohydrate: 24.3g| Protein: 32g| Fat: 25.5g

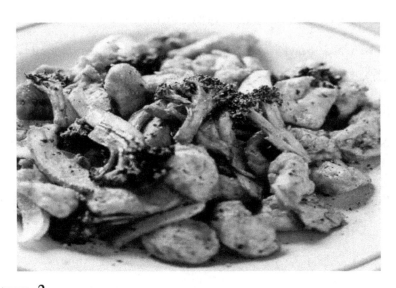

Serves: 2

Ingredients

- 1 pound of chicken, boneless & bite-size pieces
- 1-1/2 cup of broccoli
- 2 tablespoons of Grapeseed oil
- 1/3 teaspoon of garlic powder
- 1 teaspoon of ginger and garlic paste
- 2 teaspoons of soy sauce
- 1 tablespoon of sesame seed oil
- 2 teaspoons rice vinegar
- Salt and black pepper, to taste
- Oil spray, for coating

Directions

1. Take a small bowl and whisk together Grape seed oil, ginger and garlic paste, sesame seeds oil, rice vinegar, and soy sauce.

2 Take a large bowl and mix chicken pieces with the prepared marinade.

1. Let it sit for 1 hour.

2. Now, slightly grease the broccoli with oil spray and season it with salt and black pepper.

3. Put the broccoli and chicken into the basket of the air fryer that is greased with oil spray.

4. Set it to AIR FRY mode at 390 degrees F, for 22 minutes.

5. After 8 minutes of cooking, press the START/PAUSE button and takes out the broccoli.

6. Keep continuing with the chicken cooking process.

7. Once the cooking time completes, take out the chicken and serve it with the broccoli.

Nutritional Information Per Serving: Calories588 | Fat 32.1g| Sodium457mg | Carbs 4g | Fiber1.3 g | Sugar 1g | Protein67.4 g

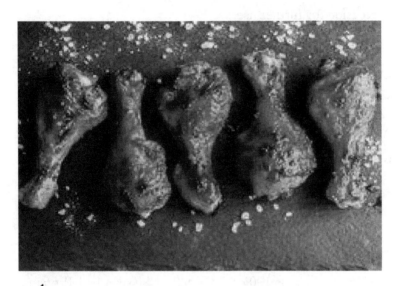

Serves: 1

Ingredients

- 1 teaspoon of onion powder

- 1 teaspoon of paprika powder

- 1 teaspoon of garlic powder

- Salt and black pepper, to taste

- 1 tablespoon of Italian seasoning

- 1 teaspoon of celery seeds

- 2 eggs, whisked

- 1/3 cup buttermilk

- 1 cup of cornflour

- 1 pound of chicken leg

Directions

1. Take a bowl and whisk egg along with pepper, salt, and buttermilk.

2. Set it aside for further use.

3. Mix all the spices in a small separate bowl.

4. Dredge the chicken in egg wash then dredge it in seasoning.

5. Coat the chicken legs with oil spray.

6. At the end dust it with the cornflour.

7. Put the leg pieces into the air fryer basket.

8. Set it to 400 degrees F, for 25 minutes.

9. Let the air fryer do the magic.

Nutritional Information Per Serving: Calories 1511| Fat 52.3g| Sodium615 mg | Carbs 100g | Fiber 9.2g | Sugar 8.1g | Protein 154.2g

Spiced Chicken and Vegetables

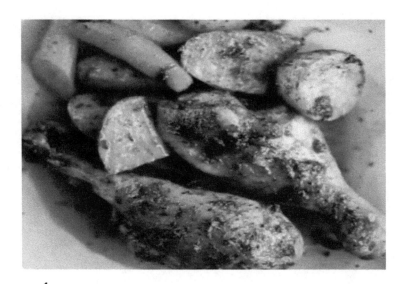

Serves: 1

Ingredients

- 2 large chicken breasts
- 2 teaspoons of olive oil
- 1 teaspoon of chili powder
- 1 teaspoon of paprika powder
- 1 teaspoon of onion powder
- ½ teaspoon of garlic powder
- 1/4 teaspoon of Cumin
- Salt and black pepper, to taste

Vegetable Ingredients

- 1 large potato, cubed

- 4 large carrots cut into bite-size pieces

- 1 tablespoon of olive oil

- Salt and black pepper, to taste

Directions

1. Take chicken breast pieces and rub olive oil, salt, pepper, chili powder, onion powder, cumin, garlic powder, and paprika.

2. Season the vegetables with olive oil, salt, and black pepper.

3. Now put the chicken breast pieces along with vegetables inside the air fryer basket.

4. Now set it to AIR FRY mode at 390 degrees F, for 35 minutes.

5. Once the cooking cycle is done, serve, and enjoy...

Nutritional Information Per Serving: Calories1510 | Fat 51.3g| Sodium525mg | Carbs 163g | Fiber24.7 g | Sugar 21.4g | Protein 102.9

Cornish Hen with Baked Potatoes

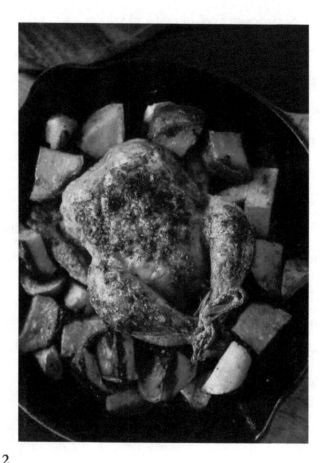

Serves: 2

Ingredients

- Salt, to taste

- 1 large potato

- 1 tablespoon of avocado oil

- 1.5 pounds of Cornish hen, skinless and whole

- 2-3 teaspoons of poultry seasoning, dry rub

Directions

1. Take a fork and pierce the large potato.

2. Rub the potato with avocado oil and salt.

3. Now put the potatoes in the bottom of the basket.

4. Now pick the Cornish hen and season the hen with poultry seasoning (dry rub) and salt.

5. Remember to coat the whole Cornish hen well.

6. Now place the hen over the potatoes inside the basket.

7. Now set it to AIR FRY mode at 350 degrees F, for 45 minutes.

8. Once the cooking cycle complete, turn off the air fryer and take out the potatoes and Cornish hen from the air fryer basket.

9. Serve hot and enjoy.

Nutritional Information Per Serving: Calories 612 | Fat14.3 g| Sodium304mg | Carbs33.4 g | Fiber 4.5 g | Sugar 1.5g | Protein 83.2 g

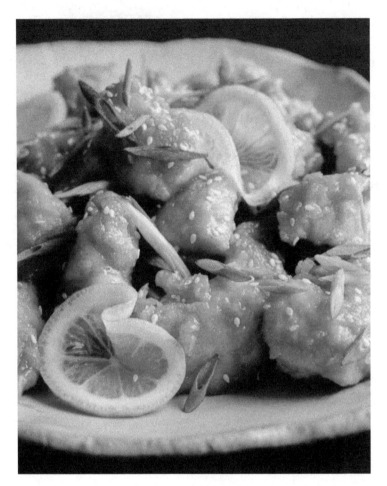

Serves: 8

Ingredients:

- 1 whole chicken

- 10 wolfberries

- 2 red chilies; chopped

- 4 ginger slices

- 1 yam; cubed

- 1 tsp. soy sauce

- 3 tsp. sesame oil

- Salt and white pepper to the taste

Directions:

1. Season chicken with salt, pepper, rub with soy sauce and sesame oil, and stuff with wolfberries, yam cubes, chilies, and ginger.

2. Place in your air fryer, cook at 400 °F, for 20 minutes, and then at 360 °F, for 15 minutes. Carve chicken, divide among plates and serve.

Nutrition Facts (Per Serving): Calories: 320; Fat: 12; Fiber: 17; Carbs: 22; Protein: 12

Devilled Eggs Nicoise

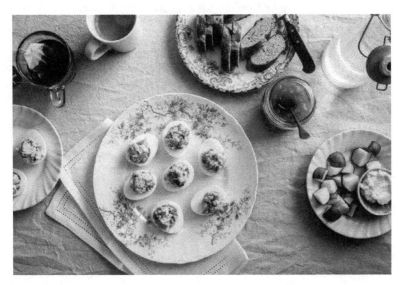

Serves: 6

Ingredients:

- 6 eggs

- 2 tablespoons black olives, minced

- 1 small tomato, seeded and minced

- 1 teaspoon Dijon mustard

- Juice of 1 lemon

- 1 tablespoon olive oil

- 1 tablespoon plain Greek yogurt

- 2 tablespoons fresh parsley, minced, plus more for garnish

Directions:

1. Preheat water bath to 170°F.

2. Place eggs in a bag. Seal with water Directions, then place in the bath. Cook for 1 hour.

3. Place eggs in a bowl of cold water to cool. Peel carefully, then cut each egg in half lengthwise.

4. Scoop egg yolks into a bowl. Stir in olives, tomato, mustard, lemon, oil, yogurt, and parsley.

5. Fill egg whites with the egg yolk mixture. Garnish with parsley.

Calories: 160, Fat 12.38g, Carbohydrates 2.59 g, Protein 9.33 g

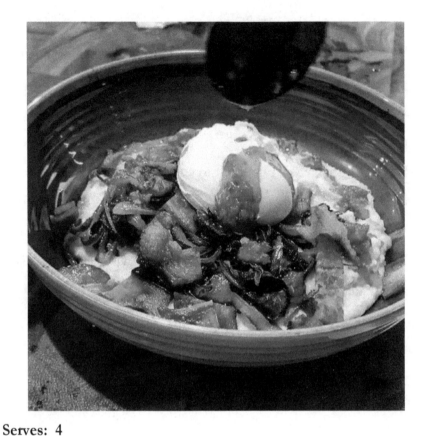

Serves: 4

Ingredients:

- 1 cup old-fashioned grits

- ½ cup plain Greek yogurt

- ½ cup milk

- 3 cups chicken stock

- 2 tablespoons butter, melted

- 4 ounces Cheddar cheese, grated, plus more for garnish

- 6 eggs

Directions:

1. Preheat water bath to 180°F.

2. Whisk together grits, yogurt, milk, stock, butter, and cheese, then pour into bag and seal using water Directions.

3. Place in a water bath and cook 2 to 3 hours, occasionally massaging to prevent lumps.

4. When the grits have ½ hour left to cook, place eggs in a bag and add to the water bath.

5. When the grits have absorbed most of the liquid, divide between 3 bowls. Carefully shell eggs and top each bowl with 2 eggs. Garnish with grated cheese.

Calories: 444, Fat 28.47 g, Carbohydrates 21.02 g, Protein 25.23 g

Huevos Rancheros

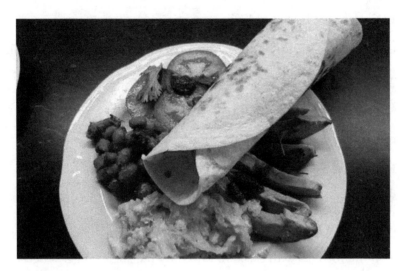

Serves: 3

Ingredients:

- ½ can (7 ounces) crushed tomatoes

- ½ small yellow onion, minced 2 cloves garlic, minced

- ¼ teaspoon dried oregano

- ¼ teaspoon ground cumin

- Juice of ½ lime

- 1 canned chipotle adobo chile, minced

- ½ can refried beans

- 6 eggs

- 6 corn tortillas

- ¼ cup fresh cilantro, chopped

- ½ cup crumbled cotija cheese or grated Monterey Jack

Directions:

1. Preheat water bath to 147°F.
2. Combine tomatoes, onion, garlic, oregano, cumin, lime, and chile in a bag. Seal using water Directions. Pour refried beans into a second bag and seal using water Directions. Place eggs into a third bag and seal using water Directions.
3. Place all three bags into the water bath. Cook for 2 hours.
4. When the other components have 20 minutes left to cook, heat tortillas in a pan. Place 2 on each plate.
5. Top the tortillas with salsa, followed by the shelled eggs, cheese, and cilantro. Serve with refried beans.

Calories: 554, Fat 34.66 g, Carbohydrates 32.71, g, Protein 28.57 g

Bar-Style Pink Pickled Eggs

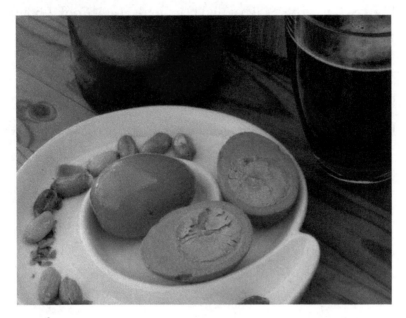

Serves: 6

Ingredients:

- 6 eggs
- 1 cup white vinegar
- Juice from 1 can beets
- ¼ cup sugar
- ½ tablespoon salt
- 2 cloves garlic
- 1 tablespoon whole peppercorn
- 1 bay leaf

Directions:

1. Preheat water bath to 170 °F.

2. Place eggs in a bag. Seal bag and place in the bath. Cook 1 hour.

3. After 1 hour, place eggs in a bowl of cold water to cool and carefully peel. In the bag in which you cooked the eggs, combine vinegar, beet juice, sugar, salt, garlic, and bay leaf.

4. Replace eggs in a bag with pickling liquid. Replace in a water bath and cook 1 additional hour.

5. After 1 hour, move eggs with pickling liquid to the refrigerator.

6. Allow cooling completely before eating.

Calories: 166, Fat 10.08 g, Carbohydrates 7.34 g, Protein 9.3 g

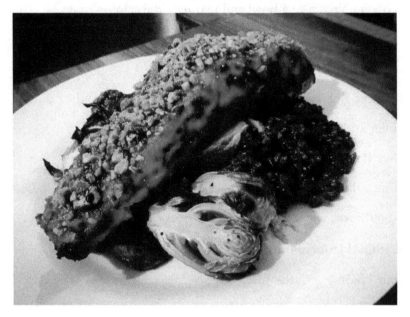

Serves: 2

Ingredients

- Oil spray, for greasing

- 2 salmon fillets, 6ounces each

- Salt and ground black pepper, to taste

- 1 tablespoon butter, for frying

- 1 tablespoon red curry paste

- 1 cup of coconut cream

- 2 tablespoons fresh cilantro, chopped

- 1 cup of cauliflower florets

- ½ cup Parmesan cheese, hard

Directions

1. Take a bowl and mix salt, black pepper, butter, red curry paste, coconut cream in a bowl and marinate the salmon in it.

2. Oil sprays the cauliflower florets and then seasons it with salt and freshly ground black pepper.

3. Put the florets in the air fryer basket and then place the salmon fillet aside.

4. Set it to AIR FRY mod at 12 minutes for4 00 degrees F

5. Once the time for cooking is over, serve the salmon with cauliflower floret with Parmesan cheese drizzle on top.

Nutritional Information Per Serving: Calories 774 | Fat 59g| Sodium1223mg | Carbs 12.2g | Fiber 3.9g | Sugar5.9 g | Protein53.5 g

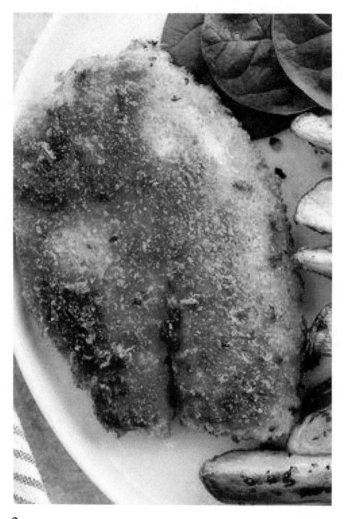

Serves: 2

Ingredients

- 4 Frozen Breaded Fish Fillet
- Oil spray, for greasing

- 1 cup mayonnaise

Directions

1. Take the frozen fish fillets out of the bag and place them in the basket of the air fryer.

2. Lightly grease it with oil spray.

3. Set the unit to 380 degrees F fo12 minutes at AIR FRY mode.

4. Hit the start button to start cooking.

5. Once the cooking is done, serve the fish hot with mayonnaise.

Nutritional Information per Serving: Calories 921 | Fat 61.5g | Sodium1575mg | Carbs 69g | Fiber 2g | Sugar 9.5g | Protein 29.1g

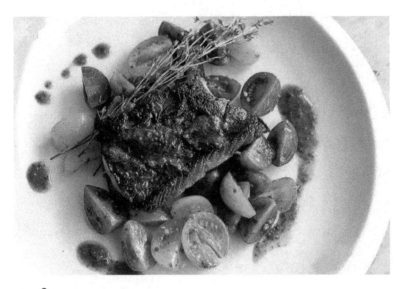

Serves: 2

Ingredients Vinaigrette Ingredients

- 1/2 cup parsley leaves

- 1 cup basil leaves

- ½ cup mint leaves

- 2 tablespoons thyme leaves

- 1/4 teaspoon red pepper flakes

- 2 cloves of garlic

- 4 tablespoons of red wine vinegar

- ¼ cup of olive oil

- Salt, to taste

Other Ingredients

- 1.5 pounds fish fillets, codfish

- 2 tablespoons olive oil

- Salt and black pepper, to taste

- 1 teaspoon of paprika

- 1teasbpoon of Italian seasoning

Directions

1. Blend the entire vinaigrette ingredient in a high-speed blender and pulse into a smooth paste.

2. Set aside for drizzling overcooked fish.

3. Rub the fillets with salt, black pepper, paprika, Italian seasoning, and olive oil.

4. Put it in the basket of the air fryer.

5. Set it to 16 minutes at 390 degrees F, at AIR FRY mode.

6. Once done, serve the fillets with the drizzle of blended vinaigrette

Nutritional Information Per Serving: Calories 1219| Fat 81.8g| Sodium1906mg | Carbs64.4 g | Fiber5.5 g | Sugar 0.4g | Protein 52.1g

Beer Battered Fish Fillet

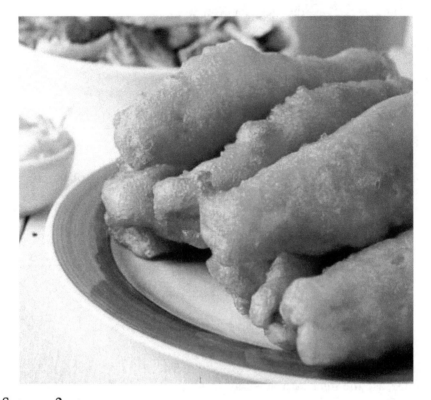

Serves: 2

Ingredients

- 1 cup all-purpose flour

- 4 tablespoons cornstarch

- 1 teaspoon baking soda

- 8 ounces beer

- 2 egg beaten

- ½ cup all-purpose flour

- 1 teaspoon smoked paprika

- 1 teaspoon salt

- 1/4 teaspoon freshly ground black pepper

- ¼ teaspoon of cayenne pepper

- 2 cod fillets, 1½-inches thick, cut into 4 pieces

- Oil spray, for greasing

Directions

1. Take a large bowl and combine flour, baking soda, corn starch, and salt

2. In a separate bowl beat eggs along with the beer.

3. In a shallow dish mix paprika, salt, pepper, and cayenne pepper.

4. Dry the codfish fillets with a paper towel.

5. Dip the fish into the eggs and coat it with seasoned flour.

6. Then dip it in the seasoning.

7. Grease the fillet with oil spray.

8. Put the fillets in the air fryer basket.

9. Set it to AIR FRY mode at 400 degrees F for 14 minutes.

10. Press start and let the AIR fry do its magic.

11. Once cooking is done, serve the fish.

Nutritional Information Per Serving: Calories 1691| Fat 6.1g| Sodium3976mg | Carbs105.1 g | Fiber 3.4g | Sugar15.6 g | Protein 270g

Chinese Cod Fillets

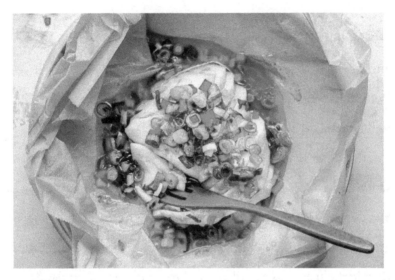

Serves: 4

Ingredients:

- 4 cod fillets, boneless

- Salt and black pepper to taste

- 1 cup water

- 4 tablespoons light soy sauce

- 1 tablespoon sugar

- 3 tablespoons olive oil + a drizzle

- 4 ginger slices

- 3 spring onions, chopped

- 2 tablespoons coriander, chopped

Directions:

1. Season the fish with salt and pepper, then drizzle some oil over it and rub well.

2. Put the fish in your air fryer and cook at 360 degrees F for 12 minutes.

3. Put the water in a pot and heat up over medium heat; add the soy sauce and sugar, stir, bring to a simmer, and remove from the heat.

4. Heat a pan with the olive oil over medium heat; add the ginger and green onions, stir, cook for 2-3 minutes, and remove from the heat.

5. Divide the fish between plates and top with ginger, coriander, and green onions.

6. Drizzle the soy sauce mixture all over, serve, and enjoy!

Nutrition: calories 270, fat 12, fiber 8, carbs 16, protein 14

Quinoa Brussels Sprout Salad

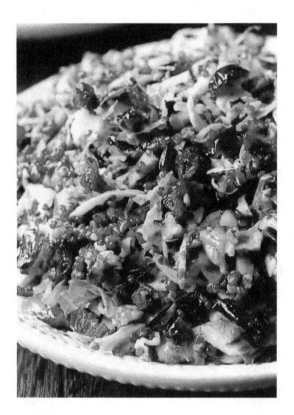

Serves: 4

Ingredients

- ½ cup cabbage, chopped

- ½ cup quinoa, rinsed

- ½ carrot, peeled and shredded

- ¾ cup water

- ¼ teaspoon salt

- 1 cup Brussels sprout, diced

- ½ cup red onions, sliced

- 1 tablespoon brown sugar

- 2 tablespoons, balsamic vinegar

- 1 tablespoon vegetable oil

- 1 tablespoon sunflower seeds

- 1 teaspoon ginger, grated

- 1 garlic clove, minced

- Black pepper to taste

Directions

1. Add the quinoa, salt, and water to the Air Fryer.

2. Secure the lid and select the "Manual" function with high pressure for 1 minute.

3. After the beep, do a quick release and remove the lid.

4. Meanwhile, add the remaining ingredients to a bowl and mix them well.

5. Add the cooked quinoa to the prepared mixture and stir.

6. Serve as a salad.

Nutrition Values (Per Serving): Calories: 151, Carbohydrate: 22.5g, Protein: 4.4g, Fat: 5.2g

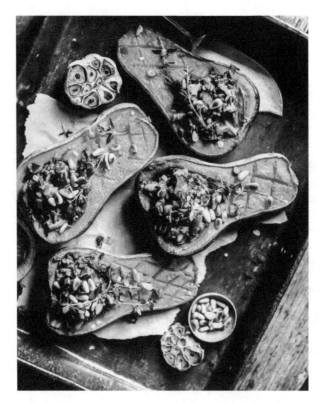

Serves: 4

Ingredients

- 1 tablespoon olive oil

- ½ cup onion, chopped

- 3 garlic cloves, minced

- 1 red bell pepper, diced

- 2 cups butternut squash, peeled and diced

- 1 ½ cups Arborio rice*

- 3 ½ cup vegetable broth

- 2 teaspoons ground coriander

- ½ cup dry white wine

- 8 oz. white mushrooms, sliced

- 1 teaspoon salt

- 1 teaspoon black pepper

- ¼ teaspoon oregano

- 1 ½ a tablespoon nutritional yeast

Directions

1. Put the oil to the insert of the Air Fryer and select the "Sauté" function.

2. Add the onion, bell pepper, butternut squash, and garlic to the oil and sauté for 5 minutes.

3. Now stir in rice, broth, salt, pepper, mushrooms, oregano, coriander, and wine.

4. Secure the lid and select the "Bean" function with 30 minutes of cooking time.

5. After the beep, do a natural release for 10 minutes then remove the lid.

6. Add the nutritional yeast, cook for another 5 minutes on the "Sauté" setting.

7. Serve warm.

Nutrition Values (Per Serving): Calories: 422, Carbohydrate: 72g, Protein: 14.5g, Fat: 5.5g

Seasoned Potatoes

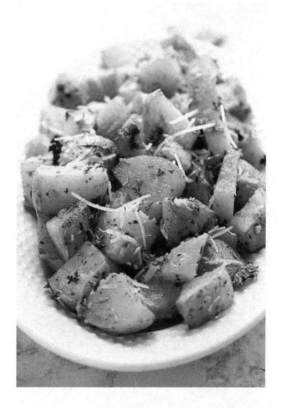

Serves: 6

Ingredients

- ½ cup avocado oil

- 3 lbs. russet potatoes, diced

- 1 teaspoon onion powder

- 2 teaspoons garlic powder

- 2 teaspoons sea salt

- ½ teaspoon paprika

- ½ teaspoon ground black pepper

- 2 cups chicken broth

Directions

1. Add the oil to the insert of the Air Fryer and select the "Sauté" function on it.

2. Add the diced potatoes, and onion to the oil and sauté for 8 minutes.

3. Now stir in all the remaining ingredients.

4. Secure the lid and select the "Manual" function with 10 minutes of cooking time.

5. After the beep, do a "Quick release" and remove the lid.

6. Sprinkle additional seasoning on top and serve.

Nutrition Values (Per Serving): Calories: 200, Carbohydrate: 38.2g, Protein: 5.9g, Fat: 3.1g

Maple-glazed Brussels Sprouts

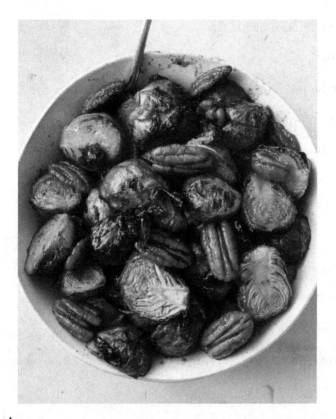

Serves: 4

Ingredients

- 1 lb. Brussels sprouts (trimmed)

- 2 tablespoons freshly squeezed orange juice

- ½ teaspoon grated orange zest

- ½ tablespoon Earth Balance buttery spread

- 1 tablespoon maple syrup

- Salt, and black pepper to taste

Directions

1. Add all the ingredients to the Air Fryer.
2. Secure the lid and select the "Manual" function for 4 minutes with high pressure.
3. Do a quick release after the beep then, remove the lid.
4. Stir well and serve immediately.

Nutrition Values (Per Serving): Calories: 166, Carbohydrate: 14.5g, Protein: 3.9g, Fat: 11.4g

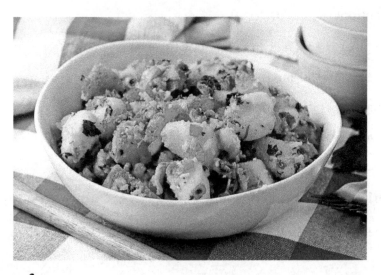

Serves: 3

Ingredients

- 3 medium russet potatoes, peeled and cubed

- 1 cup water

- 3 large eggs

- 1/8 cup finely chopped onion

- ½ cup mayonnaise

- 1 tablespoon finely chopped fresh parsley

- ½ tablespoon dill pickle juice

- ½ tablespoon mustard

- Salt and pepper to taste

Directions

1. Pour a cup of water into the insert of the Air Fryer and place the steamer trivet inside.

2. Arrange the potatoes and eggs over the trivet.

3. Secure the lid and select the "Manual" function with high pressure for 4 minutes.

4. After the beep, do a quick release and remove the lid.

5. Meanwhile, in a separate bowl combine onion, mayo, mustard, parsley, and pickle juice.

6. Add the cooked potatoes and mix gently with the mixture.

7. Peel all the eggs and dice to add to the mixture.

8. Sprinkled seasoning on top and serve.

Nutrition Values (Per Serving): Calories: 383, Carbohydrate: 44.7g, Protein: 10.8g, Fat: 18.8g

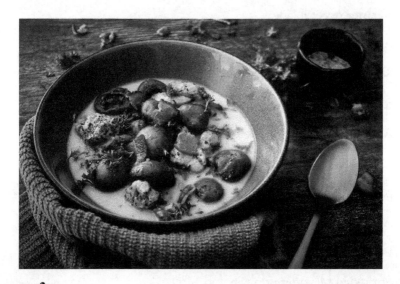

Serves: 3

Ingredients

- ½ tablespoon olive oil

- ½ lb fresh cremini mushrooms, stemmed and quartered

- ½ small onion, chopped

- ½ tablespoon tomato paste

- 1½ garlic cloves, minced

- 4 (5-oz) skinless chicken thighs

- ½ cup green olives pitted and halved

- 1 cup fresh cherry tomatoes

- ¼ cup low-sodium chicken broth

- Freshly ground black pepper to taste

- ¼ cup fresh parsley, chopped

Directions

1. Place the oil, onion, and mushrooms into the Air Fryer and cook on the 'sauté' function for 5 minutes.

2. Stir in the tomato paste, along with the garlic, and cook for another minute.

3. Add the broth, chicken, olives, and tomatoes to the pot, then secure the lid.

4. Set the 'manual' function to high pressure for 10 minutes cooking time.

5. After the beep, 'Quick release' the steam and remove the lid.

6. Sprinkle some black pepper and parsley on top.

7. Serve immediately.

Nutrition Values (Per Serving): Calories: 423, Carbohydrate: 7.8g, Protein: 57.6g, Fat: 16.7g

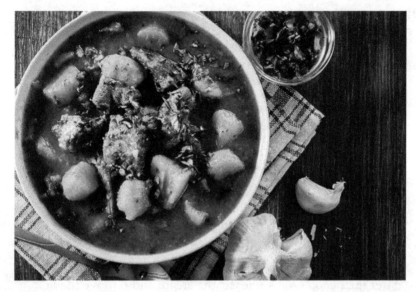

Serves: 4

Ingredients

- 1½ tablespoons olive oil

- 1½ lb. chuck roast, trimmed and cubed

- 1 cup homemade tomato sauce • ½ teaspoon smoked paprika

- 1 cup low-sodium chicken broth

- 1 large onion, cut into bite-sized pieces

- ½ lb. carrots, peeled and cut into bite-sized pieces

- ½ lb. potatoes, peeled and cut into bite-sized pieces

- ½ garlic clove, minced

- ¼ cup fresh cilantro to garnish, chopped

Directions

1. Put the oil and beef into the Air Fryer and cook on the 'sauté 'function for 5 minutes.

2. Stir in the paprika, broth, and tomato sauce, then secure the lid.

3. Cook on 'manual' settings at high pressure for 15 minutes.

4. Once done, 'quick release' the steam pressure, then remove the lid.

5. Add all the vegetables and re-lock the lid. Cook for another 20 minutes at high pressure on 'manual' settings.

6. 'Quick release' the steam, remove the lid and add the cilantro.

7. Serve immediately.

Nutrition Values (Per Serving): Calories: 320, Carbohydrate: 21.6g, Protein: 26.9g, Fat: 13.7g

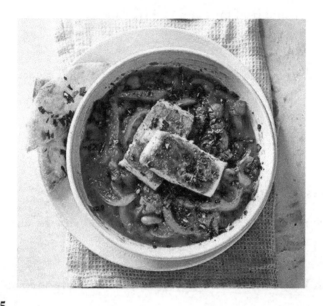

Serves: 5

Ingredients

- 1 tablespoon olive oil

- ½ carrot, peeled and minced

- ½ celery stalk, minced

- ½ small onion, minced

- 1 garlic clove, minced

- ½ teaspoon dried sage, crushed

- ½ teaspoon dried rosemary, crushed

- 4 oz. fresh Portabella mushrooms, sliced

- 4 oz. fresh white mushrooms, sliced

- ¼ cup red wine

- 1 Yukon Gold potato, peeled and chopped

- ¾ cup fresh green beans, trimmed and chopped

- 1 cup tomatoes, chopped

- ½ cup tomato paste

- ½ tablespoon balsamic vinegar

- 1¼ cups water

- 1 tablespoon corn starch

- ⅛ cup water

- Salt and freshly ground black pepper to taste

- 2 oz. frozen peas

Directions

1. Select the 'sauté' function on your Air Fryer and pour in the oil. Add the celery, carrot, and onion. Cook for 3 minutes.

2. Add the herbs and garlic to the pot and cook for another minute.

3. Now add the mushrooms and sauté for 5 minutes. Stir in the wine and cook for 2 minutes.

4. Add the green beans, potatoes, tomato paste, tomatoes, water, and vinegar, and secure the lid.

5. Set to high pressure in the 'manual' function for 15 minutes. When finished, 'quick release' the steam.

6. Combine the corn starch with water in a separate bowl to make a slurry.

7. Remove the lid of the cooker and add the corn starch slurry, peas, black pepper, and salt.

8. Cook for 1 minute on the 'sauté' setting; transfer to a bowl and serve hot.

Nutrition Values (Per Serving): Calories: 197, Carbohydrate: 36.9g, Protein: 6.6g

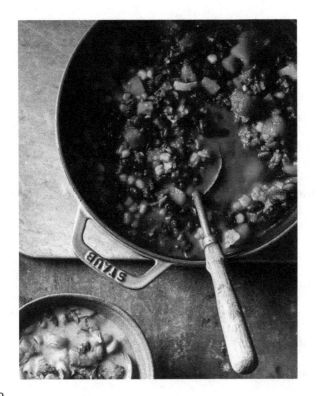

Serves: 8

Ingredients

- 1 tablespoon olive oil

- 2 lbs. ground beef

- 1 onion, chopped

- 1 green bell pepper, seeded and chopped

- 2 garlic cloves, minced

- 1 teaspoon dried oregano, crushed

- 3 tablespoons red chili powder

- 1 tablespoon ground cumin

- 3½ cups tomatoes, chopped finely

- 1½ cups cooked red kidney beans

- 1½ cups water

- ½ cup sour cream

Directions

1. Place the oil and the beef in the Air Fryer and cook for 5 minutes on the 'sauté' function.

2. Once cooked, transfer the beef to a plate.

3. Add all the vegetables and stir fry for 5 minutes.

4. Add the beef and all the remaining ingredients, except the sour cream, then secure the lid.

5. Cook on the 'manual' function for 10 minutes at high pressure.

6. Once done, 'Quick release' the steam and then remove the lid.

7. Serve with sour cream topping.

Nutrition Values (Per Serving): Calories: 769, Carbohydrate: 96.4g, Protein: 67.3g, Fat: 14.6g

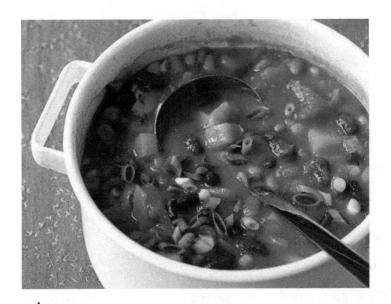

Serves: 4

Ingredients

- 1 tablespoon olive oil

- 1 cup onion, chopped

- ½ green bell pepper, seeded and chopped

- ½ cup carrot, peeled and chopped

- 2 tablespoons celery stalk, chopped

- ½ tablespoon garlic, minced

- ¼ dried kidney beans, rinsed, soaked for 8 hours and drained

- ¼ cup dried pinto beans, rinsed, soaked for 8 hours, and drained

- ¼ cup dried black beans, rinsed, soaked for 8 hours, and drained

- 1 cup fresh tomatoes, chopped

- 1 cup homemade tomato paste

- 1 teaspoon dried oregano, crushed

- 1 tablespoon mild chili powder

- ½ teaspoon smoked paprika

- ½ teaspoons ground cumin

- ¼ teaspoon ground coriander

- 2 cups low-sodium vegetable broth

- Scallions to garnish, chopped

Directions

1. Select the 'sauté' function on the Air Fryer, add the oil, bell pepper, celery, onion, carrot and garlic, and cook for 5 minutes.

2. Add the remaining ingredients to the pot then secure the lid.

3. Select the 'manual' function and set to high pressure. Cook for 15 minutes.

4. After the beep, use the 'natural release' function to vent the steam, then remove the lid. 5. Garnish with scallion and serve.

Nutrition Values (Per Serving): Calories: 282, Carbohydrate: 50g, Protein: 13g, Fat: 4.7g

Fudge Brownies

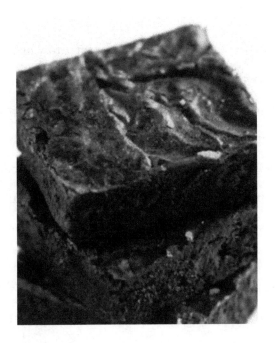

Serves: 4

Ingredients

- 1/2 cup all-purpose flour

- 1/4 cup unsweetened cocoa powder

- 3/4 teaspoon kosher salt

- 2 large eggs, whisked

- 1 tablespoon almond milk

- 1/2 cup brown sugar

- 1/2 cup packed white sugar

- 1/2 tablespoon vanilla extract

- 8 ounces of semisweet chocolate chips, melted

- 2/4 cup unsalted butter, melted

Directions

1. Take a medium bowl, and use a hand beater to whisk together eggs, milk, both the sugars, and vanilla.

2. In a separate microwave-safe bowl, mix melted butter and chocolate and microwave it for 30 seconds to melt the chocolate.

3. Add all the listed dry ingredients to the chocolate mixture.

4. Now incorporate the egg bowl ingredient into the batter.

5. Spray a reasonable size round baking pan that fits in the basket of air fryers.

6. Grease the pan with cooking spray.

7. Now pour the batter into the pan, put the crisper plate in the basket.

8. Add the pan and insert the basket into the unit.

9. Select the AIR FRY mode and adjust the set temperature to 300 degrees F, for 30 minutes.

10. Check it after 35 minutes and if not done, cook for 10 more minutes

11. Once it's done, take it out and let it get cool before serving.

Nutritional Information Per Serving: Calories 760| Fat43.3 g| Sodium644 mg | Carbs 93.2g | Fiber5.3 g | Sugar 70.2g | Protein 6.2g

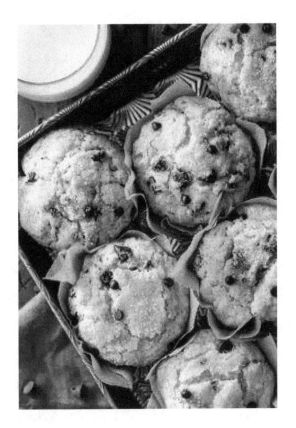

Serves: 2

Ingredients

- Salt, pinch
- 2 eggs
- 1/3 cup brown sugar
- 1/3 cup butter
- 4 tablespoons of milk
- ¼ teaspoon of vanilla extract

- ½ teaspoon of baking powder

- 1 cup all-purpose flour

- 1 pouch chocolate chips, 35 grams

Directions

1. Take 4 oven-safe ramekins that are the size of a cup and layer them with muffin papers.

2. In a bowl, whisk the egg, brown sugar, butter, milk, and vanilla extract.

3. Whisk it all very well with an electric hand beater.

4. Now, in a second bowl, mix the flour, baking powder, and salt.

5. Now, mix the dry ingredients slowly into the wet ingredients.

6. Now, at the end fold in the chocolate chips and mix them well

7. Divide this batter into 4 ramekins.

8. Now, put the ramekins in the basket.

9. Set the time to 15 minutes at 350 degrees F, at AIRFRY mode.

10. Check if not done, and let it AIR FRY for one more minute.

11. Once it is done, serve.

Nutritional Information Per Serving: Calories 757 | Fat40.3g | Sodium 426mg | Carbs 85.4g | Fiber 2.2g | Sugar 30.4g | Protein 14.4g

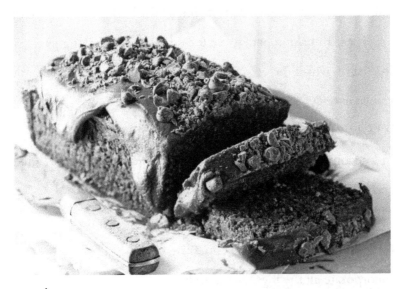

Serves: 4

Ingredients

- Salt, pinch

- 2 eggs, whisked

- ½ cup brown sugar

- ½ cup butter, melted

- 10 tablespoons of almond milk

- ¼ teaspoon of vanilla extract

- ½ teaspoon of baking powder

- 1 cup all-purpose flour

- 1 cup of chocolate chips

- ½ cup of cocoa powder

Directions

1. Take a large baking pan that fits inside the basket of the air fryer.

2. Layer it with baking paper, cut it to the size of a baking pan.

3. In a bowl, whisk the egg, brown sugar, butter, almond milk, and vanilla extract.

4. Whisk it all very well with an electric hand beater.

5. In a second bowl, mix the flour, cocoa powder, baking powder, and salt.

6. Now, mix the dry ingredients slowly with the wet ingredients.

7. Now, at the end fold in the chocolate chips.

8. Incorporate all the ingredients well.

9. Pour this batter into the round baking pan.

10. put it inside the basket.

11. Set the time to 15 minutes at 350 degrees F at AIR FRY mode.

12. Check if not done, and let it AIR FRY for one more minute.

13. Once it is done, serve.

Nutritional Information Per Serving: Calories 736| Fat45.5g| Sodium 356mg | Carbs 78.2g | Fiber 6.1g | Sugar 32.7g | Protein11.5 g

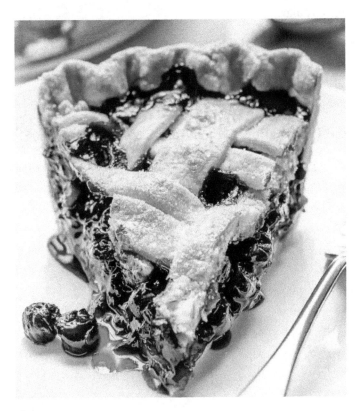

Serves: 4

Ingredients

- 1 box Store-Bought Pie Dough, Trader Joe's

- ¼ cup blueberry jam

- 1 teaspoon of lemon zest

- 1 egg white, for brushing

Directions

1. Take the store brought pie dough and cut it into 3-inch circles.

2. Brush the dough with egg white all around the parameters.

3. Now add blueberry jam and zest in the middle and top it with another circular.

4. Press the edges with the fork to seal it.

5. Make a slit in the middle of the dough and transfer it to the basket.

6. Set it to AIR FRY mode at 360 degrees for 10 minutes.

Nutritional Information Per Serving: Calories 234| Fat8.6g| Sodium187 mg | Carbs 38.2 g | Fiber 0.1g | Sugar13.7 g | Protein 2g

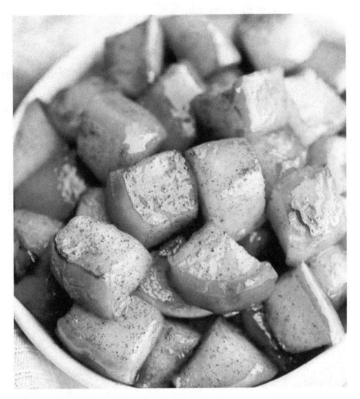

Serves: 4

Ingredients:

- 4 red apples, cored, peeled, and sliced

- 4 tbsp. butter

- 2 tsp ground cinnamon

- 2 tsp liquid honey

- Juice of 1 lemon

Directions:

1. Set your cooking device to 180 degrees F.

2. Put the ingredients into the plastic bag, and seal it, removing the air.

3. Put the bag into the Air Fryer chamber and set the cooking time for 1 hour 10 minutes.

4. Serve warm in bowls with a spoon of vanilla ice cream (optionally).

Nutrition per serving: Calories: 250, Protein: 1 g, Fats: 12 g, Carbs: 35 g

Index

B

C

D

E

Cooking Conversion Chart

TEMPERATURE		WEIGHT	
FAHRENHEIT	**CELSIUS**	**IMPERIAL**	**METRIC**
100 °F	37 °C	1/2 oz	15 g
150 °F	65 °C	1 oz	29 g
200 °F	93 °C	2 oz	57 g
250 °F	121 °C	3 oz	85 g
300 °F	150 °C	4 oz	113 g
325 °F	160 °C	5 oz	141 g
350 °F	180 °C	6 oz	170 g
375 °F	190 °C	8 oz	227 g
400 °F	200 °C	10 oz	283 g
425 °F	220 °C	12 oz	340 g
450 °F	230 °C	13 oz	369 g
500 °F	260 °C	14 oz	397 g
525 °F	270 °C	15 oz	425 g
550 °F	288 °C	1 lb	453 g

MEASUREMENT			
CUP	**ONCES**	**MILLILITERS**	**TABLESPOON**
1/16 cup	1/2 oz	15 ml	1
1/8 cup	1 oz	30 ml	3
1/4 cup	2 oz	59 ml	4
1/3 cup	2.5 oz	79 ml	5.5
3/8 cup	3 oz	90 ml	6
1/2 cup	4 oz	118 ml	8
2/3 cup	5 oz	158 ml	11
3/4 cup	6 oz	177 ml	12
1 cup	8 oz	240 ml	16
2 cup	16 oz	480 ml	32
4 cup	32 oz	960 ml	64
5 cup	40 oz	1180 ml	80
6 cup	48 oz	1420 ml	96
8 cup	64 oz	1895 ml	128

CPSIA information can be obtained
at www.ICGtesting.com
Printed in the USA
BVHW091359250521
608095BV00002B/403